Glucose Regulation

The life changing approach for optimizing blood sugar to enhance healthy living.

By

Nora R. Cooney

Table of content

I. Introduction

A. Overview of glucose metabolism

Glucose metabolism refers to the process by which cells in the body convert glucose into energy. Glucose is a simple sugar that is a major source of energy for the body's cells. The process of glucose metabolism occurs in the mitochondria and involves several metabolic pathways including glycolysis, citric acid cycle, and oxidative phosphorylation. During glycolysis, glucose is converted into pyruvate, which can be further metabolized to produce energy. The citric acid cycle and oxidative phosphorylation are two additional pathways that generate energy from glucose. These pathways produce ATP, which is the energy currency of the cell. When the body needs energy, glucose is taken up by cells and metabolized to provide the energy needed for cellular processes. Imbalances in glucose metabolism can lead to diseases such as diabetes.

B. The significance of glucose regulation

The regulation of glucose levels in the body is important for several reasons:

Energy supply: Glucose is the primary source of energy for the body, and proper regulation of glucose levels ensures that the body has a constant supply of energy for various functions.

Homeostasis: Maintaining stable glucose levels is critical for maintaining the overall balance, or homeostasis, of the body. Abnormal glucose levels can disrupt this balance, leading to health problems.

Diabetes: Impaired regulation of glucose levels is a hallmark of diabetes, a disease in which the body is unable to effectively regulate glucose levels.

Insulin secretion: The regulation of glucose levels is closely linked to insulin secretion. Insulin, a hormone produced by the pancreas, helps regulate glucose levels by facilitating its uptake into cells.

Metabolic processes: Proper regulation of glucose levels is essential for many metabolic processes, such as glycolysis, citric acid cycle, and oxidative phosphorylation.

In summary, the regulation of glucose levels plays a crucial role in maintaining the energy balance, homeostasis, and proper functioning of the body. Disruptions in glucose regulation can have serious consequences for health.

C. Purpose of the book

The purpose of the book "The Glucose Revolution" is to provide information and understanding of the role of glucose (sugar) in human metabolism and health, and to advocate for a diet and lifestyle based on stabilizing blood sugar levels through the consumption of foods that produce a low glycemic response. The book argues that this approach can lead to improved health outcomes and the prevention or management of certain health conditions such as diabetes, obesity, heart disease, and others.

II. Understanding Glucose Metabolism

A. Definition of Glucose

Glucose is a simple sugar (monosaccharide) that is an important source of energy for living organisms. It is a six-carbon molecule with the chemical formula $C_6H_{12}O_6$. Glucose is found in many foods, and is also produced by the body through the breakdown of carbohydrates. In the human body, glucose is the primary source of energy for the cells and is transported through the bloodstream.

There are three forms of glucose:

D-glucose: also known as dextrose, this is the most common form of glucose and is found in many foods.

L-glucose: a mirror image of D-glucose, this form is not commonly found in nature and is not used as a source of energy by the body.

Alpha-glucose: this is a stereoisomer of D-glucose that occurs in some complex carbohydrates and is not commonly found in nature.

B. Anatomy of Glucose Metabolism

Glucose metabolism is the process by which glucose, a type of sugar, is converted into energy for the body to use. It occurs in several steps:

Absorption: Glucose is absorbed into the bloodstream from the small intestine after a meal.

Transport: Glucose is transported into cells by insulin, a hormone produced by the pancreas.

Glycolysis: Inside the cells, glucose is broken down into pyruvate through a process called glycolysis. This releases energy in the form of ATP (adenosine triphosphate).

Aerobic respiration: If enough oxygen is available, pyruvate is further broken down into carbon dioxide and water, releasing even more energy. This process is called aerobic respiration.

Anaerobic respiration: If oxygen is not available, pyruvate is converted into lactic acid through a process called anaerobic respiration. This releases energy, but also causes muscle fatigue and pain.

Energy production: The energy produced through glucose metabolism is used by cells to perform various functions, such as muscle contraction and nerve transmission.

Storage: Any unused glucose is stored as glycogen in the liver and muscle tissue, to be used later as needed.

Overall, glucose metabolism is an important process for providing energy to the body, and it is regulated by hormones such as insulin and glucagon.

C. The Role of Insulin in Glucose Metabolism

Insulin plays a crucial role in regulating glucose metabolism in the body. It is a hormone produced by the pancreas that helps to control the level of glucose in the blood. When glucose enters the bloodstream after a meal, insulin signals the cells to absorb and store the excess glucose, mainly as glycogen in the liver and muscle tissue. Insulin also promotes the uptake of glucose into fat cells, where it can be stored for later use as energy. At the same time, insulin inhibits the production and release of glucose by the liver and also stimulates the conversion of glucose into fats. In this way, insulin helps to regulate blood glucose levels and ensure a steady supply of energy for the body's needs.

D. Factors that Affect Glucose Regulation

The factors that affect glucose regulation in the human body include:

Insulin secretion: Insulin secretion by the pancreas regulates glucose levels in the blood by promoting glucose uptake into cells and suppressing glucose production by the liver.

Hormonal signals: Hormonal signals from the gut and liver play a role in regulating glucose levels, such as glucagon from the pancreas and epinephrine from the adrenal glands.

Physical activity: Physical activity increases glucose uptake by muscles, which can lower glucose levels in the blood.

Food intake: The consumption of carbohydrates, particularly simple sugars, can raise glucose levels in the blood.

Stress: Physical or psychological stress can cause the release of stress hormones, such as cortisol and epinephrine, which can affect glucose regulation.

Sleep: Sleep patterns and disruptions can affect glucose regulation.

Age and gender: As people age, their insulin sensitivity may decline, affecting glucose regulation, and hormones related to glucose regulation may vary between men and women.

Chronic diseases: Chronic diseases, such as obesity and type 2 diabetes, can affect glucose regulation and insulin sensitivity.

III. Glucose Disorders

Glucose disorder refers to a group of medical conditions related to the regulation of glucose levels in the blood. Glucose is the primary source of energy for the body and its level must be kept within a narrow range to ensure proper functioning of the body.

The types of glucose disorder included:

A. Hypoglycemia

Hypoglycemia is a medical condition characterized by low blood sugar levels, typically below 70 mg/dL. It occurs when the body has an insufficient amount of glucose, which is the primary source of energy for the brain and body. Common symptoms of hypoglycemia include weakness, fatigue, shakiness, sweating, confusion, irritability, and hunger. Severe cases can lead to unconsciousness and seizures.

Hypoglycemia can be caused by a number of factors, including an overproduction of insulin, skipping a meal, consuming too much alcohol, or engaging in physical activity without eating enough food. People with diabetes who take insulin or oral medications that increase insulin levels are at a higher risk for hypoglycemia.

Treatment for hypoglycemia involves eating or drinking a source of fast-acting sugar, such as fruit juice, candy, or glucose gel. It is important to monitor blood sugar levels and have a plan in place for treating hypoglycemia. Long-term management may involve adjusting medications, modifying diet and exercise habits, and working with a healthcare provider to develop a customized plan.

If you suspect that you or someone you know is experiencing hypoglycemia, it is important to seek medical attention promptly. With proper management, most people with hypoglycemia are able to maintain normal blood sugar levels and lead healthy, active lives

B. Hyperglycemia

Hyperglycemia is a medical condition characterized by an elevated level of glucose (sugar) in the blood. It is a common symptom of uncontrolled diabetes, but can also occur in individuals who do not have diabetes. The elevated glucose levels can damage organs and tissues over time and increase the risk of developing serious health problems such as heart disease, stroke, kidney damage, nerve damage, and blindness. Symptoms of hyperglycemia include frequent urination, excessive thirst, blurred vision, fatigue, and slow healing of wounds. Treatment depends on the underlying cause, but may involve lifestyle changes such as diet modification, increased physical activity, and medication management. Regular monitoring of blood glucose levels is also important in managing hyperglycemia.

C. Insulin Resistance

This is a condition in which the body's cells begin to oppose the effectiveness of the insulin, a hormone produced by the pancreas. Insulin's main function is to regulate blood sugar levels by facilitating the uptake of glucose into cells. When cells are insulin resistant, they require more insulin than normal to perform this function, leading to higher insulin levels in the blood. Over time, this can lead to a range of health problems, including type 2 diabetes, heart disease, and stroke. The exact causes of insulin resistance are not fully understood, but it is often associated with a sedentary lifestyle, a diet high in refined carbohydrates, and being overweight or obese. Treatment typically involves lifestyle changes, such as increasing physical activity and improving the quality of one's diet, as well as medications to manage blood sugar levels.

D. Prediabetes and Type 2 Diabetes

Prediabetes and Type 2 diabetes are two conditions related to the regulation of glucose in the body. Prediabetes is a condition where by the blood sugar level is higher than normal but not high enough to be called type 2 diabetes. On the other hand, type 2 diabetes is a condition in which the body cannot produce enough insulin to regulate glucose levels, leading to high blood sugar levels.

Prediabetes is a serious health condition that often leads to type 2 diabetes if left untreated. People with prediabetes have a higher risk of developing heart disease, stroke, and other health problems. The condition is often detected by blood glucose tests and is usually diagnosed in people over the age of 45 years, overweight or obese individuals, and those with a family history of type 2 diabetes.

Type 2 diabetes is a severe condition that affects millions of people all over the world. The condition is often caused by a combination of genetics and lifestyle factors, such as poor diet, lack of physical activity, and obesity. People with type 2 diabetes have high blood sugar levels, which can lead to various health complications, including heart disease, kidney disease, blindness, and nerve damage.

Treatment for prediabetes and type 2 diabetes involves lifestyle changes, such as a healthy diet, regular exercise, and weight loss. In some cases, medicine may be necessary to monitor blood sugar levels. It is important to work with a healthcare provider to create a personalized treatment plan that works best for each individual.

In conclusion, prediabetes and type 2 diabetes are serious health conditions that affect millions of people worldwide. Regular screening, healthy lifestyle changes, and proper medical treatment can help prevent and manage these conditions, reducing the risk of related health complications. It is important to take control of one's health and seek help from healthcare providers when necessary.

E. Complications of Glucose Disorders

There are several types of glucose disorders, including diabetes, hypoglycemia, and hyperglycemia. Each of these conditions can have serious and potentially life-threatening complications if not managed properly.

Diabetes: This is a condition in which the body's ability to produce or use insulin, the hormone that regulates glucose levels in the blood, is compromised. This leads to high levels of glucose in the blood, known as hyperglycemia, which can cause serious complications if left uncontrolled. Some of the most common complications of diabetes include:

Cardiovascular disease: People with diabetes are more likely to develop heart disease and stroke, due to the damage that high glucose levels can cause to blood vessels and the heart.

Nerve damage: High glucose levels can damage the nerves in the body, leading to neuropathy, or nerve pain and numbness in the hands and feet.

Kidney damage: Diabetes can cause the kidneys to stop working properly, leading to a condition known as diabetic nephropathy. This can eventually lead to kidney failure and the need for dialysis.

Eye damage: High glucose levels can cause damage to the blood vessels in the eyes, leading to vision loss and even blindness.

Foot problems: Diabetes can cause damage to the nerves and blood vessels in the feet, making it difficult to heal from injuries and leading to foot ulcers and amputations.

Hypoglycemia: This is a condition in which the glucose levels in the blood become too low, leading to symptoms such as confusion, shakiness, sweating, and fatigue. Some of the complications of hypoglycemia include:

Seizures: Seizures can occur in people with hypoglycemia, especially if the condition is not recognized and treated quickly.

Coma: In severe cases of hypoglycemia, the brain can be affected, leading to confusion, unconsciousness, and coma.

Increased risk of falls: Hypoglycemia can cause dizziness, confusion, and unsteadiness, increasing the risk of falls and injury.

Hyperglycemia: This is a condition in which the glucose levels in the blood become too high, leading to symptoms such as frequent urination, excessive thirst, and blurred vision. Some of the complications of hyperglycemia include:

Dehydration: High glucose levels can cause excessive thirst, leading to dehydration and an increased risk of kidney problems.

Infections: High glucose levels can make it difficult for the body to fight off infections, increasing the risk of serious infections such as pneumonia and urinary tract infections.

Coma: In severe cases of hyperglycemia, the brain can be affected, leading to confusion, unconsciousness, and coma.

In conclusion, glucose disorders can have serious and potentially life-threatening complications if not managed properly. It is important for people with these conditions to work closely with their healthcare provider to ensure that they are taking the appropriate steps to manage their condition and reduce their risk of complications.

IV. Glucose Management

Glucose management refers to the process of monitoring and controlling the levels of glucose (sugar) in the bloodstream. This is important for people with diabetes and those at risk of developing the disease, as high levels of glucose in the bloodstream can lead to serious health problems.

People with type 1 diabetes are unable to produce insulin, a hormone that helps regulate blood sugar levels. Those with type 2 diabetes either produce insufficient insulin or their bodies are unable to use it effectively. In both cases, glucose management involves taking steps to keep blood sugar levels within a safe range.

Effective glucose management starts with monitoring blood sugar levels regularly. This can be done using a blood glucose meter, which measures the amount of glucose in a small drop of blood. People with diabetes are typically advised to check their blood sugar levels several times a day, especially before and after meals.

Diet and exercise play a key role in glucose management. A balanced diet that includes carbohydrates, proteins, and healthy fats can help regulate blood sugar levels. Physical activity also helps to regulate glucose levels by increasing insulin sensitivity and reducing the risk of developing type 2 diabetes.

Medications and insulin injections can also be used to manage glucose levels. In some cases, oral medications can be prescribed to help regulate blood sugar levels. For people with type 1 diabetes or advanced type 2 diabetes, insulin injections may be necessary to keep glucose levels under control.

In addition to these steps, it is important for people with diabetes to regularly see a healthcare provider to monitor their glucose levels and overall health. This may include monitoring for complications such as heart disease, eye problems, and nerve damage.

In conclusion, glucose management is essential for people with diabetes and those at risk of developing the disease. Regular monitoring, a balanced diet, physical activity, and appropriate medications or insulin injections can help keep blood sugar levels within a safe range and reduce the risk of serious health problems.

A. Lifestyle Changes for Better Glucose Regulation

Lifestyle changes play a critical role in regulating glucose levels and maintaining good health for individuals with diabetes. Whether it is through diet, exercise, stress management or sleep habits, making positive changes can lead to better glucose regulation and improved overall health.

Diet: Eating a balanced, nutritious diet that is low in sugar and processed foods is essential for better glucose regulation. This means including plenty of fresh fruits and vegetables, lean protein, and healthy fats in your diet. Limiting sugary drinks such as soda and juice and replacing them with water or low-fat milk can also help regulate glucose levels.

Exercise: Frequent exercise is a relevant component for a healthy living. It can help regulate glucose levels by improving insulin sensitivity and promoting the release of insulin. Plan to exercise for at least 30 minutes per day, 5 days in a week. This can be through activities such as walking, running, cycling or even playing sports.

Stress Management: Stress can have a significant impact on glucose levels and should be managed through activities such as yoga, meditation or deep breathing exercises. You can also manage stress by taking breaks from work and engaging in activities you enjoy such as reading, cooking, or gardening.

Sleep Habits: A good night's sleep is critical for overall health and can also help regulate glucose levels. Aim to get at least 7 hours of sleep each night, and avoid caffeine, alcohol, and screens in the hours leading up to bedtime.

In conclusion, making lifestyle changes is an essential aspect of managing diabetes and regulating glucose levels. Whether it is through diet, exercise, stress management or sleep habits, these changes can lead to better glucose regulation and improved overall health.

B. Diet and Nutrition for Glucose Regulation

Diet and nutrition play a crucial role in glucose regulation, as what we eat affects the levels of glucose in our blood. These are some important points to bare in mind:

Carbohydrates: They are the main source of glucose and are broken down into glucose in the digestive system. To regulate blood glucose levels, it is important to choose carbohydrates wisely and consume them in moderate amounts. Whole grains, fruits, and vegetables are good options.

Fiber: It is an indigestible carbohydrate that slows down digestion and helps regulate blood glucose levels by preventing rapid spikes in blood glucose.

Protein: It can also impact glucose levels, as the body breaks down protein into glucose when there is not enough carbohydrate available for energy. It is important to choose lean protein sources, such as chicken, fish, and legumes, to regulate glucose levels.

Fat: It has a minimal effect on glucose levels, but it is still an important part of a healthy diet. Choose fats that are healthy, like olive oil, avocados, and nuts, and limit saturated and trans fats.

Portion control and meal timing: Eating frequent, balanced meals throughout the day can help regulate glucose levels, as can controlling portion sizes. Eating a high-carbohydrate meal can cause a rapid spike in blood glucose, so it is important to spread carbohydrate intake evenly throughout the day.

It is important to consult with a registered dietitian or a healthcare provider to tailor a diet and nutrition plan that fits individual needs and goals for glucose regulation.

C. Exercise and Physical Activity

Exercise and physical activity are critical components for maintaining glucose regulation and preventing the onset of diabetes. When we engage in physical activity, the muscles use glucose as fuel to generate energy, which helps to lower the amount of glucose in the bloodstream. In addition, exercise also stimulates the production of insulin, which helps to move glucose from the bloodstream into the cells where it can be used for energy or stored for later use.

The type of exercise you do can affect glucose regulation. Aerobic exercise, such as brisk walking, running, cycling, and swimming, is the most effective type of exercise for regulating glucose levels. This is because it raises your heart rate and increases blood flow to the muscles, which leads to an increased demand for glucose. Resistance training, such as weightlifting, can also help to regulate glucose levels, but it is not as effective as aerobic exercise.

Physical activity also has a lasting effect on glucose regulation, even after the activity has been completed. This is because exercise increases insulin sensitivity, which means that the cells become more responsive to insulin and are better able to take in glucose from the bloodstream. This improved insulin sensitivity can last for several hours after exercise, which can help to keep glucose levels under control for the rest of the day.

In addition to its effects on glucose regulation, physical activity also has a number of other health benefits, including reducing the risk of cardiovascular disease, improving mental health, and strengthening bones and muscles.

To get the most benefit from physical activity for glucose regulation, it is important to make exercise a regular part of your routine. Target at least 30 minutes of average-intensity aerobic exercise, like brisk walking, most days of the week. Resistance training can also be included as part of your routine, but it should not be used as a substitute for aerobic exercise.

In conclusion, exercise and physical activity are crucial components of a healthy lifestyle for people with diabetes or those at risk for developing the disease. Regular exercise can help to regulate glucose levels, improve insulin sensitivity, and reduce the risk of other health problems. So, make exercise a part of your daily routine and enjoy the many benefits it has to offer!

D. Medications and Treatments

There are various medications and treatments for regulating glucose levels, including:

Oral hypoglycemic agents: These medications work by increasing insulin sensitivity, reducing glucose production by the liver, or improving glucose uptake by cells. Examples include metformin, sulfonylureas, and meglitinides.

Insulin therapy: This treatment is used for individuals with type 1 diabetes or advanced type 2 diabetes who are unable to produce or properly use insulin. Insulin can be administered through injections or an insulin pump.

Incretin-based therapies: These medications mimic the effects of naturally occurring hormones in the gut that stimulate insulin production and lower glucose production by the liver. Examples include glucagon-like peptide-1 (GLP-1) receptor agonists and dipeptidyl peptidase-4 (DPP-4) inhibitors.

Bariatric surgery: This type of surgery, such as gastric bypass or sleeve gastrectomy, can lead to significant weight loss and improvement in glucose regulation for individuals with obesity and type 2 diabetes.

Lifestyle changes: Making healthy dietary choices, engaging in regular physical activity, and maintaining a healthy weight are important components of glucose regulation.

It is important to note that the best treatment plan for regulating glucose levels will depend on the individual and the underlying cause of their hyperglycemia. A healthcare professional should be consulted to determine the most appropriate treatment plan.

E. Monitoring Glucose Levels

Monitoring glucose levels is an important aspect of managing diabetes or ensuring that your blood sugar remains within a healthy range. There are several methods to monitor glucose levels, including blood glucose meters, continuous glucose monitoring systems, and laboratory tests.

Blood Glucose Meters: Blood glucose meters are the most commonly used method of monitoring glucose levels. They are small, portable devices that measure the amount of glucose in a small drop of blood. You can use these meters at home, work or anywhere else to check your glucose levels. Simply place a drop of blood on a test strip, insert it into the meter, and within seconds, the meter will display your glucose level.

Continuous Glucose Monitoring Systems: Continuous glucose monitoring systems (CGM) consist of a small sensor that is placed under the skin and a wearable device that displays glucose levels. The sensor measures glucose levels in the interstitial fluid, which is the fluid that surrounds cells in the body. CGMs can provide real-time glucose readings and alert you when your glucose levels are too high or too low.

Laboratory Tests: Laboratory tests such as hemoglobin A1c (HbA1c) and fasting plasma glucose (FPG) are also used to monitor glucose levels. HbA1c provides an average of your glucose levels over the past 2 to 3 months. FPG is a blood test that measures glucose levels after an overnight fast. These tests are typically performed by a healthcare provider and provide a comprehensive overview of your glucose levels.

Regardless of the method you choose, monitoring glucose levels regularly is crucial in maintaining healthy blood sugar levels. It allows you to make necessary adjustments to your diet, exercise, and medication regimen, and helps you avoid complications associated with uncontrolled diabetes.

In conclusion, monitoring glucose levels is a critical aspect of managing diabetes or ensuring that your blood sugar remains within a healthy range. There are several methods to monitor glucose levels, including blood glucose meters, continuous glucose monitoring systems, and laboratory tests. Speak to your healthcare provider to determine the best method for you.

V. Natural Approaches to Glucose Regulation

A. Herbs and Supplements for Glucose Control

Herbs and supplements are sometimes used to help control blood sugar levels. However, it is important to note that they may not have been thoroughly tested and their effects can vary greatly among individuals. Some of the popular herbs and supplements that are believed to have an impact on glucose control are:

Cinnamon: It is believed to improve insulin sensitivity and reduce blood sugar levels.

Chromium: It is an essential mineral that may help improve insulin sensitivity and glucose metabolism.

Bitter Melon: It is a tropical fruit that has been used traditionally for blood sugar control and is thought to improve insulin sensitivity.

Alpha-Lipoic Acid: It is an antioxidant that may improve insulin sensitivity and glucose uptake by the cells.

Gymnema Sylvestre: It is an herb commonly used in Ayurvedic medicine that is thought to improve insulin sensitivity and reduce blood sugar levels.

It's important to consult with a doctor before taking any herbs or supplements as they can interact with medications and cause adverse effects. Additionally, they may not be suitable for everyone and should not be used as a substitute for a balanced diet and regular physical activity, which are the best ways to maintain healthy blood sugar levels.

B. Mind-Body Techniques for Glucose Regulation

Mind-body techniques, such as meditation, yoga, and deep breathing, have been found to help regulate glucose levels in the body. These techniques work by reducing stress and promoting relaxation, which in turn can help to stabilize blood sugar levels. When the body is under stress, cortisol and other hormones are released, causing an increase in blood sugar. By reducing stress, mind-body techniques can help to mitigate this response and maintain healthy glucose levels.

In addition to reducing stress, mind-body techniques can also improve insulin sensitivity, which is the body's ability to use insulin effectively to regulate blood sugar levels. For example, research has shown that regular practice of yoga can lead to improved insulin sensitivity, which can help to lower blood sugar levels.

Overall, incorporating mind-body techniques into a lifestyle that includes a healthy diet and regular exercise can be an effective way to help regulate glucose levels and maintain overall health. However, it's important to note that these techniques should not be considered a replacement for medical treatment or advice from a healthcare provider.

C. The Role of Sleep and Stress in Glucose Metabolism

Sleep and stress are important factors that affect glucose metabolism, which is the process by which the body converts food into energy.

Sleep deprivation can disrupt glucose metabolism and increase insulin resistance, making it harder for the body to regulate blood sugar levels. As a result, there is a high chance of developing type 2 diabetes. Adequate sleep is essential for maintaining healthy glucose metabolism and preventing the onset of metabolic disorders.

Stress can also have a significant impact on glucose metabolism. Chronic stress increases cortisol levels, which can lead to elevated blood sugar levels and decreased insulin sensitivity. This can increase the risk of developing type 2 diabetes, especially in people who are already predisposed to the disease.

In addition, stress can also interfere with the normal functioning of the HPA axis, which is responsible for regulating cortisol levels. This can lead to further disruption of glucose metabolism, making it important to manage stress levels in order to maintain healthy glucose metabolism.

Overall, the role of sleep and stress in glucose metabolism is significant and highlights the importance of maintaining a healthy sleep pattern and managing stress levels in order to maintain healthy glucose metabolism and prevent the onset of metabolic disorders.

D. Integrative Approaches to Glucose Management

Integrative approaches to glucose management involve a holistic approach to managing glucose levels. This approach takes into account the interplay of physical, emotional, and lifestyle factors that impact glucose levels. It involves combining traditional medical treatments with complementary and alternative therapies to achieve optimal glucose control.

One of the key components of integrative approaches to glucose management is lifestyle modification. This includes changes in diet, exercise, and stress management. A balanced diet that is low in processed foods and high in fiber and nutrient-rich whole foods can help regulate glucose levels. Exercise, such as regular physical activity and resistance training, can also help regulate glucose levels and improve insulin sensitivity.

Stress management techniques, such as mindfulness and relaxation practices, can help reduce the impact of stress on glucose levels.

Complementary and alternative therapies, such as acupuncture, massage, and herbal remedies, can also play a role in integrative approaches to glucose management. For example, acupuncture has been shown to improve insulin sensitivity and glucose uptake in people with type 2 diabetes. Herbal remedies, such as cinnamon, fenugreek, and gymnema, can also help regulate glucose levels and improve insulin sensitivity.

VI. Conclusion

A. The Importance of Optimal Glucose Regulation

Glucose regulation is a crucial aspect of human health, as it determines the amount of energy available for bodily functions and helps prevent various diseases. Optimal glucose regulation refers to maintaining a stable blood glucose level, which is essential for good health. The following are some of the reasons why optimal glucose regulation is so important.

Prevention of diabetes: Optimal glucose regulation helps prevent the development of type 2 diabetes, a condition where the body is unable to regulate glucose levels effectively. People with uncontrolled glucose levels are at a higher risk of developing type 2 diabetes, which can lead to serious health problems such as heart disease, nerve damage, and kidney damage.

Improved energy levels: Optimal glucose regulation helps ensure that the body has enough energy available to carry out its daily activities. When glucose levels are too high or too low, the body is unable to function optimally, and people may feel tired, sluggish, or irritable.

Better mental health: Optimal glucose regulation has been linked to improved mental health, as fluctuations in glucose levels can affect mood, energy levels, and cognitive function. People with uncontrolled glucose levels are more likely to experience anxiety, depression, and other mental health problems.

Better physical health: Optimal glucose regulation helps prevent the development of various physical health problems, including heart disease, stroke, and kidney damage. People with uncontrolled glucose levels are also more likely to experience complications from other health conditions, such as infections, skin problems, and vision problems.

Long-term health benefits: Optimal glucose regulation can lead to long-term health benefits, including a reduced risk of developing chronic diseases, improved mental and physical well-being, and a longer lifespan.

In conclusion, optimal glucose regulation is essential for good health, and people should strive to maintain stable glucose levels through healthy lifestyle choices, such as regular exercise, a balanced diet, and stress management. People with uncontrolled glucose levels should seek medical advice to prevent the development of serious health problems.

B. The Power of Knowledge and Action

The power of knowledge and action in glucose regulation is vital for maintaining a healthy body. Glucose is the primary source of energy for our cells and it's regulated by hormones such as insulin and glucagon. When our blood glucose levels rise, the pancreas releases insulin to stimulate the uptake of glucose by cells and its storage as glycogen. On the other hand, when blood glucose levels fall, glucagon signals the liver to break down glycogen into glucose and release it into the bloodstream.

Having a good understanding of glucose regulation and how it is influenced by various factors such as diet, physical activity, and medication is crucial in managing conditions such as diabetes. By taking appropriate actions, individuals with diabetes can maintain optimal glucose levels, prevent long-term complications, and lead a healthy and active life.

For example, incorporating physical activity into your daily routine and following a balanced diet can help regulate glucose levels, while avoiding sugary and processed foods can prevent spikes in blood glucose. Regular monitoring of glucose levels and taking insulin injections or oral medications as prescribed can also greatly impact glucose regulation.

In conclusion, the power of knowledge and action in glucose regulation plays a crucial role in maintaining a healthy body and preventing long-term complications. By taking the right steps and working with a healthcare provider, individuals with diabetes can lead a healthy and active life.

C. Achieving Optimal Glucose Balance

Achieving optimal glucose balance involves maintaining stable blood sugar levels, which can be done through several methods:

Eating a balanced diet: This includes consuming foods that are high in fiber, protein, and healthy fats, and reducing the intake of processed and sugary foods.

Exercising regularly: Physical activity can help lower blood sugar levels and increase insulin sensitivity.

Monitoring blood sugar levels: Regular monitoring of blood sugar levels can help individuals understand how different foods, activities, and medications impact their levels.

Taking medications as prescribed: For individuals with diabetes, taking medications such as insulin or oral hypoglycemic agents as prescribed by a healthcare professional is important in managing blood sugar levels.

Reducing stress: Stress can impact blood sugar levels and thus it's important to find ways to manage stress effectively.

Getting enough sleep: Getting adequate sleep helps regulate hormones that impact glucose levels.

It's important to consult with a healthcare professional to determine the best approach for achieving optimal glucose balance, as individual needs may vary.

D. Final Thoughts and Recommendations.

Final Thoughts on Glucose Regulation:

Glucose regulation is an essential aspect of overall health and wellness. Imbalances in glucose levels can lead to a variety of health problems, including diabetes, obesity, and heart disease. To maintain optimal glucose regulation, it is important to make lifestyle changes, such as regular exercise, a balanced diet, and stress management.

Recommendations for Glucose Regulation:

Exercise: Regular physical activity can help regulate glucose levels and reduce the risk of developing diabetes. Target at least 30 minutes of less intense exercise a day.

Healthy Diet: Incorporate fiber-rich foods, such as fruits and vegetables, into your diet to help regulate glucose levels. Limit your intake of processed foods and sugar.

Stress Management: Chronic stress can disrupt glucose regulation. Practice stress management techniques, such as mindfulness, deep breathing, and yoga, to help regulate glucose levels.

Monitor Glucose Levels: Regularly check your glucose levels to stay informed of any changes. Keep a log of your readings and share them with your healthcare provider.

Medications: If necessary, take medications as prescribed by your healthcare provider to regulate glucose levels.

In conclusion, glucose regulation is an important aspect of overall health and wellness. By making lifestyle changes, such as regular exercise, a balanced diet, and stress management, you can help regulate glucose levels and reduce the risk of developing related health problems. Always seek the opinion of your healthcare provider before making any adjustment to your diet or exercise schedule.

www.ingramcontent.com/pod-product-compliance
Lightning Source LLC
Chambersburg PA
CBHW061558250726
48657CB00021B/2246